the essence of
aromatherapy

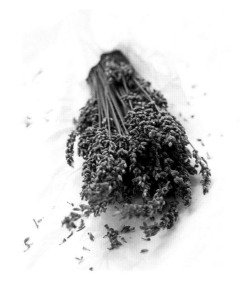

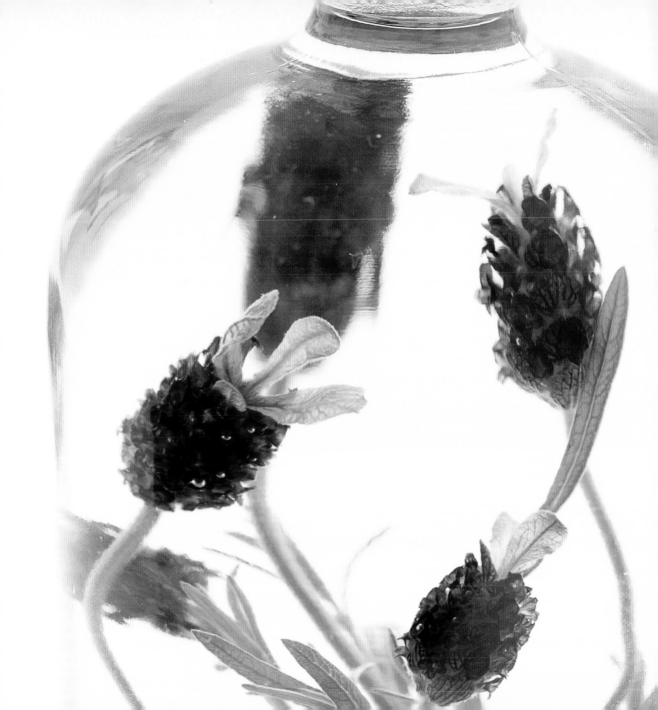

the essence of
aromatherapy

Glenda Taylor

photography by David Montgomery

RYLAND
PETERS
& SMALL
LONDON NEW YORK

Designer Vicky Holmes
Editor Maddalena Bastianelli
Location Research Sarah Hepworth
Production Patricia Harrington, David Meads
Art Director Gabriella Le Grazie
Publishing Director Anne Ryland

Stylist Serena Hanbury
Additional Photography Tom Leighton (p. 6)

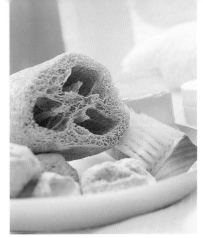

First published in the United Kingdom in 2000.
This new edition first published in 2004 by
Ryland Peters & Small
Kirkman House
12–14 Whitfield Street
London W1T 2RP
www.rylandpeters.com

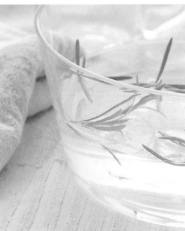

10 9 8 7 6 5 4 3 2 1

The publisher thanks Ros Fairman for allowing them to photograph in her
house, in London (pp. 28–29).

ISBN 1 84172 630 3
A CIP catalogue record for this book is available from the British Library.

Printed and bound in China

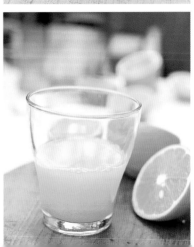

**Before using any essential oils, please read the guidelines for use
on page 15 and refer to the precautions in the essential oils chart
on pages 18–21. The applications and quality of essential oils is
beyond the control of the author and the publisher, who cannot
be held responsible for any problems arising from their use.**

contents

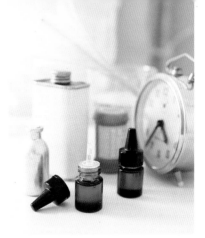

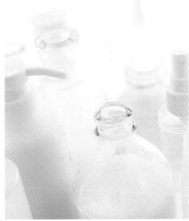

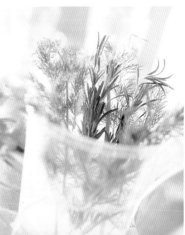

introduction

The benefits of plants in treating body and mind were known to our ancestors thousands of years ago. Now science has come full circle and we are re-discovering all that plants have to offer.

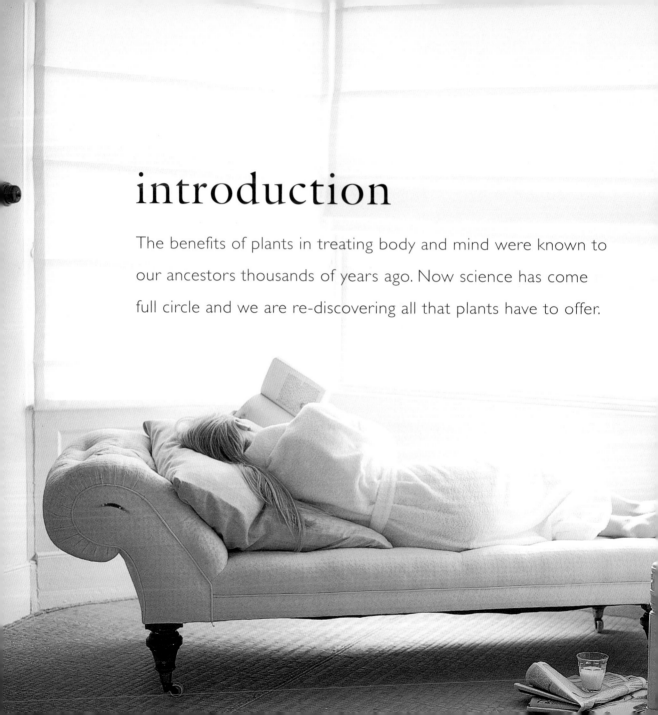

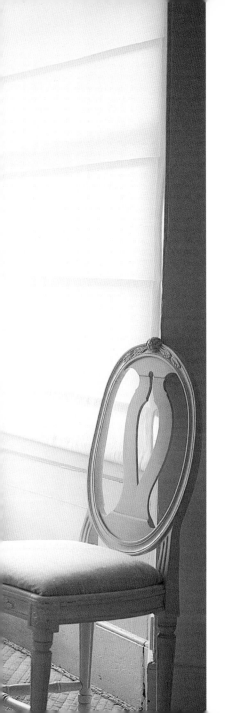

For thousands of years plants have played a vital role in medicine. Aromatherapy – using the scent of essential oils for healing – was probably first discovered by cavemen inhaling the scent of burning leaves and woods. But ancient Eygptians are regarded as the founders of aromatherapy. Archaeologists discovered that many urns excavated from tombs once contained highly prized essential oils. We also know that the ancient Greeks and Romans were advocates of them, too.

With the growth of modern medicine, natural remedies were cast aside and risked being lost for ever. Then in 1937, René Gattefosse, a French chemist, burned his hand. Relief came when he plunged it into the nearest liquid – luckily it was lavender oil. His injury healed so quickly that he decided to research the therapeutic values and properties of plant extracts.

A few years later, during the Second World War, a shortage of medication led a French surgeon, Dr Jean Valnet, to use essential oils instead. Some proved more effective than the intended drugs.

But it was an Austrian surgical assistant, Marguerite Maury in the 1950s and 60s, who shaped the aromatherapy of today. She worked on blending oils specific to the needs of the individual.

Gradually we have come full circle. Disillusionment with mainstream drugs, as well as a desire to control our own health and lives has seen a return to aromatherapy. It is effective, pleasurable and can be integrated easily into anyone's life.

the basics

understanding aromatherapy

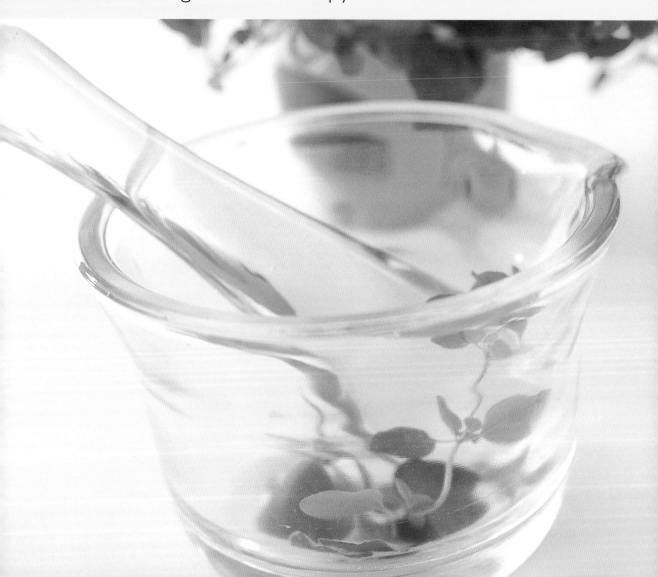

A romatherapy is a vast subject encompassing the study of the human body, plants, methods of extraction and many types of complementary therapies. It is a completely natural therapy that has many diverse uses. Its essential oils can be used as a fragrance, in bathing, for vaporizing and inhaling, or in conjunction with the powerful touch of massage and reflexology. The joy of aromatherapy is that, from the moment you take an interest in it, you can begin to apply it to treat your physical, psychological and emotional needs. You will quickly discover that aromatherapy can enhance, even shape and influence your life. Don't be afraid to try. Everyone – from newborn upwards – can benefit. Learning the intricacies of aromatherapy is a long journey and this book is just a beginning – it is the essence of aromatherapy.

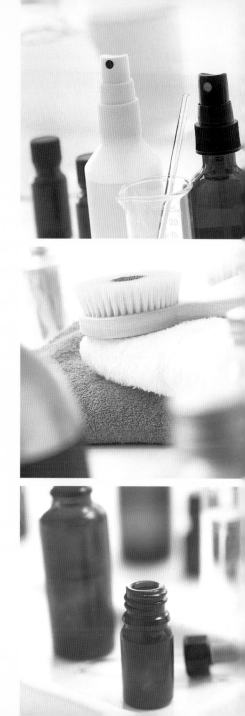

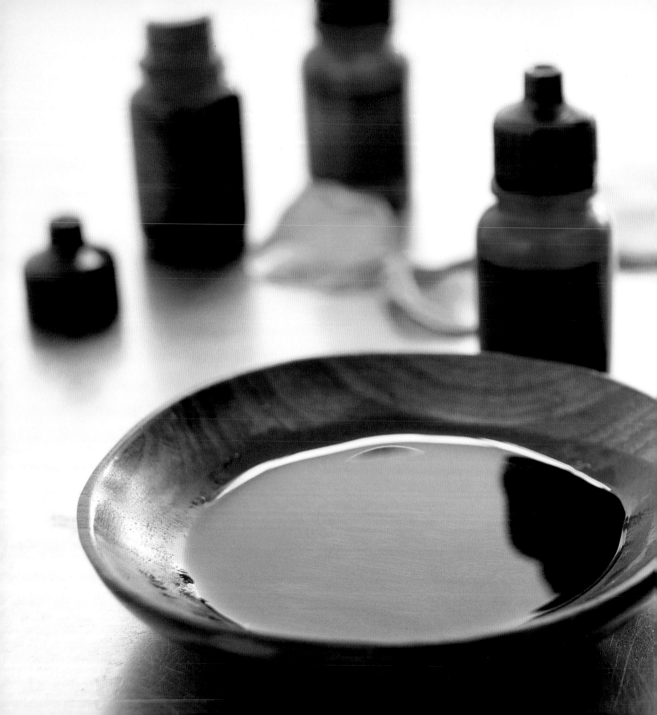

Aromatherapy is an holistic treatment that promotes overall wellbeing rather than treating an illness in isolation. It combines the sciences of chemistry and botany with the art of blending essential plant oils.

how it works

The healing molecules of essential oils enter the body by inhalation or through the skin, then into the bloodstream.

There are two routes by which the essential oils enter the body: through the nose by inhalation or by absorption through the skin. When the oil is inhaled, tiny molecules are absorbed into the bloodstream via capillaries in the nose, throat and lungs. As the oil circulates around the body, it acts according to its specific properties. Some oils are stimulating or sedating, others antibacterial, and so on. This versatility makes it possible to tailor treatments to suit individual needs. The nose is also the direct pathway to the olfactory centre in the brain, so inhaling scents can influence mood and affect hormonal secretions.

Absorption through the skin is achieved primarily through massage. Tiny pores in the skin draw the oils into the capillaries and from there into the bloodstream and lymphatic system. Massage also promotes deep, relaxed breathing, so allowing the oils to be inhaled at the same time.

Using essential oils in bathing, vaporizing, inhaling, massage, neat application (only when advised), compresses and reflexology are the techniques of aromatherapy.

Finally, the benefits of aromatherapy are enhanced by a positive outlook. If you like an oil's fragrance and believe in its therapeutic powers, you will be more responsive to its overall effects.

An essential oil is a complex chemical substance extracted from aromatic plants. Its quality and properties depend on the species of the plant and the conditions it grows in. Even the time of day when the plant matter is harvested is important.

The quality and quantity of the essential oil is also affected by the way it is extracted. There are three main methods of extraction – steam distillation, expression and enfleurage.

Steam distillation is the most common method. Pressurized steam is pumped through the plant material and the resulting vapour is cooled and collected.

Expression is used to squeeze citrus oils from the fruit's peel. It is the simplest and cheapest form of essential oil production.

Enfleurage is an expensive and time-consuming process used to extract oil from fragile flowers such as rose, jasmine and neroli, whose oils evaporate if subjected to heat. Instead, the petals are coated in wax which absorbs the oil, then solvents are used to separate the two. The resulting oil is referred to as an absolute.

Delicate floral oils are the most

essential oils

Essential oils possess properties unique to their plant species. Aromatherapy harnesses these properties to help create physical and mental wellbeing.

expensive of all essential oils. It takes 100 kilos of rose petals to produce just ½ kilo of oil, whereas the same weight of eucalyptus will yield 10 kilos of essential oil.

The scent of the essential oils used in aromatherapy can trigger all sorts of emotions and memories which in turn evoke a powerful physical response in the body. But while these oils are powerful in effect, they are delicate in composition. Light, heat and oxygen make them deteriorate, so they should be kept in a cool place in tightly stoppered dark glass bottles.

Essential oils are also highly concentrated, so they must be treated with respect. Do not use them neat, unless this has been recommended to you, and never take them internally without prior professional consultation.

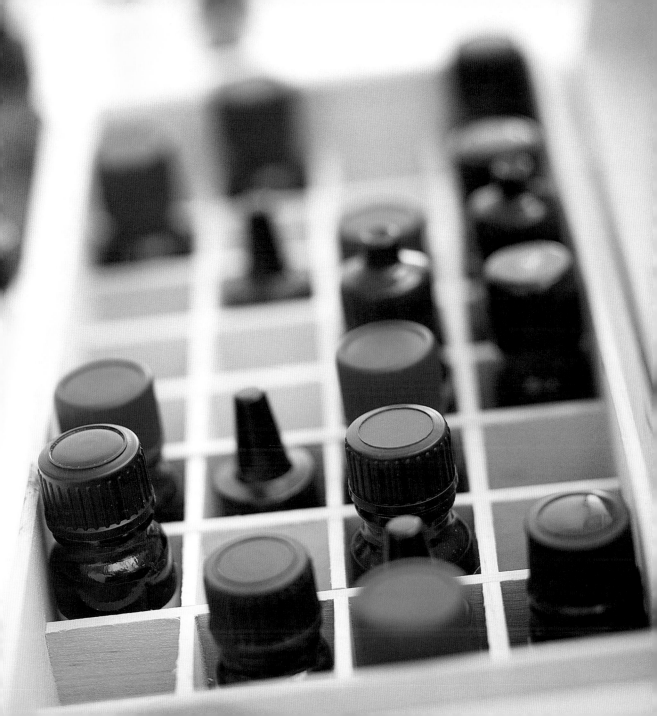

In the majority of aromatherapy skin preparations, essential oils are diluted and blended before use with neutral oils known as carrier or base oils. These oils help to disperse the essential oils, while moisturizing and conditioning the skin. Vegetable oils such as grapeseed, peach kernel or soya are perfect for

carrier oils and blending

If essential oils are to be applied to the skin, they must be blended with a neutral carrier oil. When oils are vaporized or added to a bath, air and water are the carriers.

this purpose. Oils containing vitamin E, such as jojoba, avocado, and wheat germ are sometimes blended with essential oils to make richer skin preparations, especially for dry skin conditions, or can be used

in combination with other carrier oils. The antioxidants in these rich oils also help to prolong the life of the blend.

Avoid strong-smelling carrier oils such as olive oil, as their scent interferes with that of the essential oil. Unperfumed gels, creams and lotions may also be used as carriers, though oil is the preferred medium. Don't be tempted to use synthetic oils as these prevent the absorption of essential oils and will leave your skin feeling sticky and greasy.

Perfumers divide scent into three 'notes'. Top notes are perceived first but fade quickly; middle notes are longer lasting and add richness and body to a fragrance; base notes last the longest, adding depth and fullness to the overall aroma. The same principle can be applied to essential oils in aromatherapy. Light oils such as lemon and grapefruit provide top notes; lavender, rose and geranium, middle notes; sandalwood and vetivert, the base notes.

Blending oils offers limitless possibilities for creating aromatherapy treatments and once you become familiar with the various oils, you will be able to create your own blends.

There is no need to be rigid when you are blending essential oils. It is not an exact science and one or two drops more or less will not be harmful. Using a dropper will stop you from accidentally adding the wrong amount. However, don't be tempted to add extra essential oil to increase the fragrance or effect. The warmth of your skin will bring out the aroma and a

blend which is too strong might have an unpleasant effect.

As when learning any new skill, practice makes perfect. However, for the safe and effective use of essential oils, you should follow a few basic guidelines:

● For adults with normal skin, do not exceed 5 drops of essential oil to every 10 ml (1 dessertspoon) of carrier oil.

● For babies and small children, add a maximum of 1–2 drops of essential oil to every 10 ml (1 dessertspoon) of carrier oil.

● If using essential oils with strong stimulating properties, like some citrus oils, you may want to add less essential oil to the carrier oil.

● Before applying a blend to the skin, you should carry out a patch test, especially for people with sensitive skin. Apply it first to a small area and leave for

twenty-four hours to check for any adverse or allergic reactions.

● Do not use more than five essential oils in one blend. If you do, you will compromise its aroma and effects.

● For best results, do not store blends but make them up in small quantities as and when they are needed.

below Essential oils are usually measured using an integral dropper.

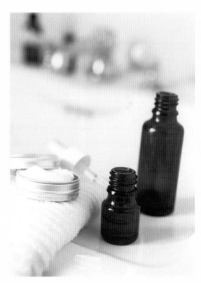

essential oils

choosing the right oil for your needs

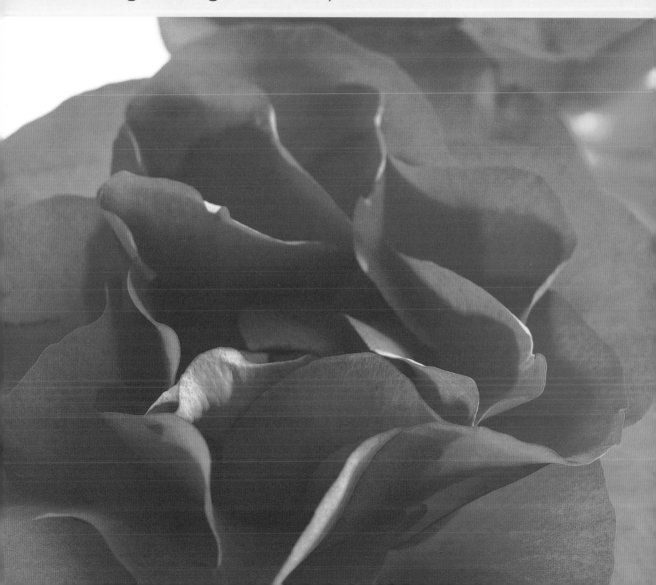

O ver a hundred essential oils are used in aromatherapy, but thankfully fewer are needed for everyday treatments. Many have similar therapeutic properties, so choosing a suitable one can be confusing. With this is mind I have compiled a chart of forty-five essential oils comprising oils for skincare preparations; for physical wellbeing; to influence moods and emotions, and much more. I have also included an indepth look at ten of the oils – my must-have 'wonder' oils – such as lavender, rose and eucalyptus with suggestions for use across all age groups. Bear in mind that mental and physical health are linked; if the scent of an essential oil conjures up pleasant associations, this psychological effect will make an unbalanced body or mind more adept at healing itself.

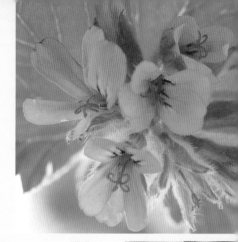
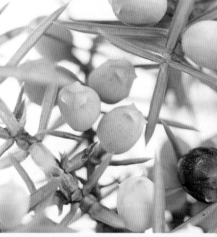
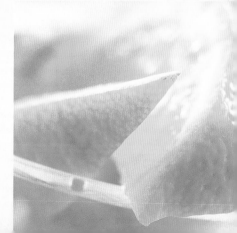

top forty-five essential oils

quick-reference guide to the healing properties of essential oils

essential oil	skincare	emotional	medicinal	precautions
basil (Ocimum basilicum)	antiseptic, especially good for spots	fortifying; stimulating; helpful for depression	treats digestive aches and pains, chest complaints and travel sickness	do not use on people with high blood pressure or epilepsy; avoid during pregnancy; not suitable for children
benzoin (Styrax benzoin)	treats chapped, dry skin	calming; eases nervous tension	treats coughs, laryngitis, aching muscles, sluggish circulation and travel sickness	can irritate sensitive skin
bergamot (Citrus bergamia)	counteracts oily skin	helpful for depression and anxiety; uplifting; mood enhancer; reviving	treats colds, coughs, sore throats and travel sickness; acts as an insect repellent	do not use before sunbathing; can irritate sensitive skin
black pepper (Piper nigrum)		fortifying; warming; appetite stimulant; increases alertness	warms aching muscles	do not use on people with high blood pressure or epilepsy; avoid during pregnancy; not suitable for children
cedarwood (Juniperus virginiana)	helps balance oily skin	settles nerves	treats aches and pains, water retention; treats scalp problems like dandruff; acts as an insect repellent	avoid during pregnancy; may irritate sensitive skin
chamomile (Anthemis nobilis)	soothes inflamed skin	calming; sedating; eases nervous tension	eases pain; treats insomnia (mild enough for babies and children)	
cinnamon (Cinnamomum zeylanicum)		combats mental exhaustion	treats chills and improves poor circulation	avoid if pregnant, suffer from high blood pressure, are epileptic or have sensitive skin; do not use for children
citronella (Cymbopogon nardus)	counteracts oily skin	refreshing; combats mental fatigue	treats colds and flu; combats fatigue; acts as an insect repellent	
clary sage (Salvia sclarea)	helps prevent oily skin	mood enhancer; calming and reassuring	treats muscular aches and pains, throat infections, hormone imbalance	avoid during pregnancy; do not use if alcohol has been consumed
clove (Eugenia caryophylla)	helps speed recovery from ulcers		soothes toothache; acts as an insect repellent	always use in weak dilutions; avoid during pregnancy
cypress (Cupressus sempervirens)	has an astringent effect on oily skin	calms nerves	treats cellulite, haemorrhoids and poor circulation	avoid during pregnancy

essential oil	skincare	emotional	medicinal	precautions
dill (Anethum graveolens)			treats flatulence (mild enough for nursing mothers); relieves colic and tummy aches in babies	
eucalyptus (Eucalyptus globulus)		clears the head; acts as a stimulant; eases mental fatigue	treats colds and flu, muscular aches and pains, wounds and insect bites	not suitable for small children or during pregnancy
fennel (Foeniculum vulgare)	brightens oily, dull skin	revitalizes; eases nervous tension	treats constipation and relieves flatulence; stimulates lactation in nursing mothers	avoid during pregnancy
frankincense (Boswellia thurifera)	relieves dry skin	deeply calming; aids concentration	treats cold and flu; revives people who are feeling run-down	
geranium (Pelargonium graveolens)	combats combination skin	mood enhancer	acts as an insect repellent; soothes tender breasts; treats cellulite, headlice and hormone imbalance	avoid during pregnancy
ginger (Zingiber officinale)		combats mental exhaustion	treats nausea, fatigue, poor circulation and indigestion	avoid during pregnancy, if suffering from high blood pressure or epilepsy; do not use with homeopathic medication
grapefruit (Citrus paradisi)	counteracts oily skin	uplifting; mood enhancer	treats cellulite, muscle fatigue and morning sickness	do not use before sunbathing
jasmine (Jasminum grandiflorum)	treats dry sensitive skin; can be used as a perfume	lifts depression; mood enhancer		
juniper (Juniperus communis)	combats oily skin	stimulates and boosts mental clarity	treats poor circulation, muscular aches and pains, rhuematism and gout; acts as a diuretic	avoid during pregnancy, if suffering from high blood pressure or if epileptic
lavender (Lavandula angustifolia)	useful for all skin types	balances and calms emotions	treats inflammation, wounds, colds and flu, cystitis, headaches, insomnia and athlete's foot	
lemon (Citrus limon)	treats very oily skin	uplifting, invigorating; clarifies thought	treats warts, cellulite, nausea, poor circulation, colds, sore throats, headlice; acts as an insect repellent	do not use before sunbathing
lemongrass (Cymbopogon citratus)	treats open pores; acts as a scalp conditioner	relieves nerves and eases stress	treats poor circulation, indigestion; breaks a fever; acts as an insect repellent	

top forty-five essential oils

quick-reference guide to the healing properties of essential oils

essential oil	skincare	emotional	medicinal	precautions
mandarin (Citrus nobilis)	reduces stretch marks and scarred oily skin	calms nerves and gently sedates; mood enchancer	eases fluid retention; aids digestion and quells stomach aches, especially in children	
marjoram (Thymus mastichina)		deeply relaxing; helpful for anxiety, stress and shock	loosens stiff muscles; eases aches, pains and arthritis; treats insomnia	avoid during pregnancy; do not use on people with low blood pressure
melissa (Melissa officinalis)		helps alleviate nervous tension; mood enhancer	aids digestion and circulation, and soothes aches and pains	a very expensive oil, comparable to rose – do not be fooled by cheap imitations
myrrh (Commiphora myrrha)	helps combat chapped, dry skin	calms and soothes nerves	treats thrush, chilblains, athlete's foot and coughs; promotes healthy circulation	avoid during pregnancy
myrtle (Myrtus communis)	counteracts oily skin	eases mental fatigue; promotes calm, even breathing	treats coughs and colds and eases congestion (mild enough for children)	
neroli (Citrus aurantium)	good for sensitive and mature skin; reduces scarring; can be used as a perfume	helps grief; reduces anxiety; helps relieve post-natal and menopausal depression	promotes healthy circulation; eases palpitations; helps prevent and treat stretch marks	
niaouli (Melaleuca viridiflora)	helps relieve oily skin	revives and refreshes	decongests colds, flu and bronchial ailments; treats aches and pains; promotes healthy circulation	avoid during pregnancy; do not use for babies and children under two years old
orange (Citrus sinensis)	helps relieve oily skin	enhances concentration; helps relieve stress and calm nerves	helps reduce and treat cellulite; eases constipation	do not use before sunbathing
palmarose (Cymbopogon martinii)	beneficial for all skin types	soothes nerves; relieves mental exhaustion	calms stomach disorders; treats wounds	
parsley (Petroselinum sativum)			aids digestion; eases flatulence; treats cellulite	avoid during pregnancy
patchouli (Pogostemon patchouli)	beneficial for all skin types	helps treat stress and nervous exhaustion	helps to relieve dermatitis, eczema and skin sores; acts as an insect repellent	

essential oil	skincare	emotional	medicinal	precautions
peppermint (Mentha piperita)		revives and boosts a tired mind; calms nerves	aids digestion and helps relieve nausea; eases headaches, treats colds and flu; soothes muscular pain	do not use with homeopathic medication; avoid during the first three months of pregnancy
petitgrain (Citrus aurantium)	combats oily skin	helps relieve stress and nervous exhaustion; mood enhancer	calms indigestion and muscular tension	
pine (Pinus pumilia)		helps relieve stress and nervous exhaustion; calms nerves	eases breathing, especially for colds, flu and asthma; eases muscular aches and pains; helps reduce excessive perspiration	
rose (Rosa centifolia)	good for mature, dry and sensitive skin; can be used as a perfume	helps lift the spirit and enhance moods; helps with grief; promotes sensual feelings	relieves hay fever and asthma; eases PMT, period pain and menopausal problems; stimulates circulation	
rosemary (Rosmarinus officinalis)	combats greasy skin	stimulates the mind to combact mental exhaustion and fatigue	useful for treating rheumatism; gets rid of headlice; stimulates circulation and relieves colds and flu	avoid during pregnancy; do not use on people suffering from high blood pressure or epilepsy
rosewood (Aniba rosaeodora)	useful for combination skin	helps calm and relieve stress	helps combat perspiration; soothes headaches; relieves nausea, especially travel sickness; treats skin infections	
sandalwood (Satalum album)	moisturizes dry skin	helps ease depression; can be used to create a sensual atmosphere	calms nausea; eases cystitis	
tea tree (Melaleuca alternifolia)	treats spots and acne		treats athlete's foot, verrucas, cold sores, spots, acne, insect bites, thrush, colds and flu	
thyme (Thymus vulgaris)	helpful for oily skin	strengthens and restores vitality	treats aches and pains, laryngitis, sore throats, tonsillitis, colds and flu; treats cellulite; improves circulation	avoid during pregnancy; do not use on people suffering from high blood pressure or epilepsy
vetivert (Vetiveria zizanioides)	counteracts oily skin	helps lift depression and relaxes the mind	eases arthritis, rheumatism, stiff joints and muscles; soothes aches and pains	
ylang ylang (Cananga odorata)	useful for combination skin	acts as a powerful aphrodisiac	eases palpitations	has a very powerful, heady aroma, so only use a little at a time

lavender
Lavandula angustifolia

There are many varieties of lavender, but *Lavandula angustifolia* is the most commonly used in aromatherapy. The word lavender comes from the Latin *lavare*, to wash, and it does indeed have a cleansing effect on both body and mind. When sleep eludes you and you can't unwind because of 'mind chatter', a drop of lavender oil dotted onto a handkerchief and placed on your pillow so you can inhale its vapours, will instantly soothe and relax. For babies, a drop of lavender oil diluted in 5 ml (1 teaspoon) of milk, then added to bathwater will calm and protect against germs, too.

Lavender's calming effect is also useful during the day – when stress levels may be high, or if you are feeling anxious, depressed or run-down. Vaporize the oil in a burner. Not only will this sedate, it will also scent the room and cleanse the air.

Interestingly, lavender's balancing properties make it a stimulant as well as a sedative. To relieve exhaustion, use the oil in the same way as above.

With antiseptic, painkilling and antibacterial properties, lavender oil is one of the few essential oils that can be used neat. A drop of oil applied directly to spots, cuts, stings, insect bites or burns will cleanse and heal them. It is also successful for treating sunburn; add a few drops of oil to a warm bath to soothe the pain. Always add the oil after the water has been run to gain full benefit.

Among lavender's many attributes is its synergistic properties, which means the oil can be blended easily

The most versatile and best-loved of all essential oils, with calming, soothing, healing and balancing properties.

with other oils (see pages 14–15) for use in massage and it can be used in massages specially for babies.

Naturally repellent to insects, lavender oil can be used to protect clothes and linens during storage. A lavender-scented handkerchief laid in a drawer or tied around a coat hanger will keep moths away.

Lavender's unique scent has been treasured for centuries, especially by the Romans who used it in bathing. Now it is fashionable again, matching today's taste for a fresh, clean fragrance.

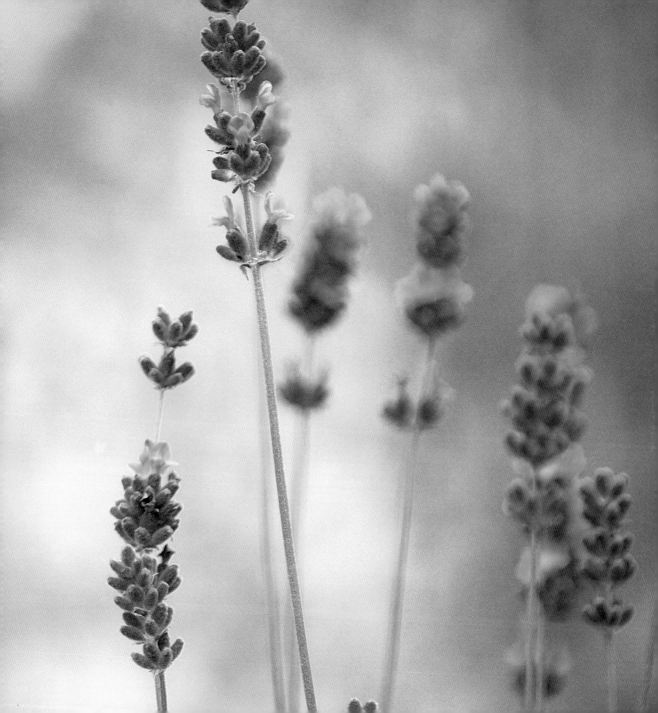

lemon *Citrus limon*

Feel invigorated, stimulated and revived by the fresh zing of lemon. It is an oil traditionally used to scent clothes and deter insects.

The fresh, sharp, tangy scent of lemon is unmistakable. This well-loved citrus fruit, grown in the Mediterranean, has been used for many years in natural home remedies – from scenting clothes to treating warts!

Like all citrus oils, lemon oil is extracted from the fruit's peel. Maximum yields of oil are obtained from the lemon when it is unripe and still green in colour.

Lemon oil has the ability to lift the spirits, open the mind and invigorate, so is invaluable first thing in the morning. Prepare for the day ahead by adding 2 drops each of lemon and rosemary oil, plus I drop each of lavender and bergamot oil to the bath or shower floor, then feel the benefits as you breathe in the oil-rich steam.

As well as having a refreshing fragrance, lemon is also antiseptic and antibacterial. Vaporizing it in a burner will help to prevent the spread of infection in a sickroom and will boost a patient's immune system.

Insects are repelled by the scent of lemon and a natural, effective deterrent can be made by vaporizing 2 drops of the oil with 2 drops each of geranium and bergamot oil.

Lemon can be useful in hair treatments too. Its insect-repellent properties can be utilized to rid headlice (see page 58), while a basic rinse of 3 drops of lemon oil diluted in a glass of warm water is good for greasy hair. Wash your hair as normal, then finish with the rinse. There is no need to wash it out, but take care not to let any get in your eyes. If this happens, rinse immediately.

Lemon oil may be used neat in only a few instances, such as in treating warts and verrucas. Use a cotton wool ball to dab a drop of oil onto the affected area twice a day. Do not use if warts are on the neck or face because the skin here is too delicate and may burn. Lemon is phototoxic, so do not use on the skin before going out in the sun, or it will have a bleaching effect.

Mandarins are named after the Chinese Mandarins who were traditionally given the fruits as gifts. They are part of the citrus family which includes orange, grapefruit, lemon, lime and bergamot and many citrus oils – extracted from the peel – are used in aromatherapy. Their general effect is euphoric and spiritually uplifting but mandarin oil has gentler and less stimulating actions, which makes it perfect for children and safe to use during pregnancy. It also has antiseptic and antispasmodic properties.

In France, mandarin oil is sometimes called the

Mild, yet highly effective: known for its gentleness and sweet, fruity fragrance.

children's oil because of its mildness and fruity fragrance. The glands in a child's stomach are very active, so illness is often accompanied by stomach ache. When a child is feeling unwell, mix 4 drops of mandarin oil and 1 drop of chamomile oil with 10 ml (1 dessertspoon) of vegetable oil and rub it onto his or her stomach. Always massage in a clockwise direction (anticlockwise will cause discomfort and will give a feeling of trapped wind).

This simple massage blend is also good during pregnancy to prevent and treat stretch marks on the stomach and buttocks. Another benefical treatment for expectant mothers is to relax in a bath scented with 3 drops of mandarin oil and 3 drops of rose oil. The effect is very soothing.

Useful in skin treatments, mandarin oil helps to reduce tissue scarring after injury by encouraging skin-cell regeneration, and because of its mild astringency, it is also effective in combating oily skin and acne. Blend 2 drops of mandarin oil and 1 drop of lavender oil with 10 ml (1 dessertspoon) of grapeseed or almond oil and gently massage a little onto your face each evening.

Mandarin oil can be used purely for its fragrance to create an atmosphere or to set a mood. It is an oil that works well in any season. In summer, when it is diffused in a vaporizer, it induces a beautifully fresh and light mood, yet in winter its scent enhances the festive atmosphere, conjuring up thoughts of the excitement of childhood Christmases. A blend of 2 drops each of mandarin, juniper and cinnamon oil releases spicy aromas when vaporized and makes this mixture a good Christmas-time choice.

mandarin

Citrus nobilis

Native to Australia, eucalyptus has strong links with the Aborigines who have used its oil for centuries as a decongestant and antiseptic. There are over 700 species of eucalyptus but only a few are used to extract essential oils. Since its discovery by Europeans, it has been widely used in traditional remedies to treat colds and

Alternatively, diffuse the blend of oils in a vaporizer, disinfecting the air at the same time as treating the illness.

As well as being one of the best decongestants, eucalyptus is a strong antiseptic preventing infection when used on minor wounds. For cuts and stings, soak a flannel in warm water with

eucalyptus *Eucalyptus globulus*

flu – to clear a blocked nose and ease breathing. The oil's instantly recognizable scent is reminiscent of soothing chest rubs. To make a chest rub, mix 2 drops of eucalyptus and myrtle oil and 1 drop of lemon oil with 10 ml of vegetable oil, then massage onto the chest, back and neck. Inhaling the vapours from a bowl of hot water containing 2 drops each of eucalyptus and peppermint oil, plus 1 drop of lemon oil is equally effective.

2 drops each of eucalyptus and lavender oil, then wring out the flannel and apply it to the affected area at regular intervals.

Eucalyptus oil is very stimulating, so do not use it on anyone who is pregnant or who suffers from high blood pressure, heart disease, hypertension or epilepsy. Instead, choose other oils with similar decongestant properties, such as niaouli, myrtle or pine. Myrtle is mild enough to use, diluted, for babies with colds.

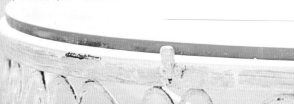

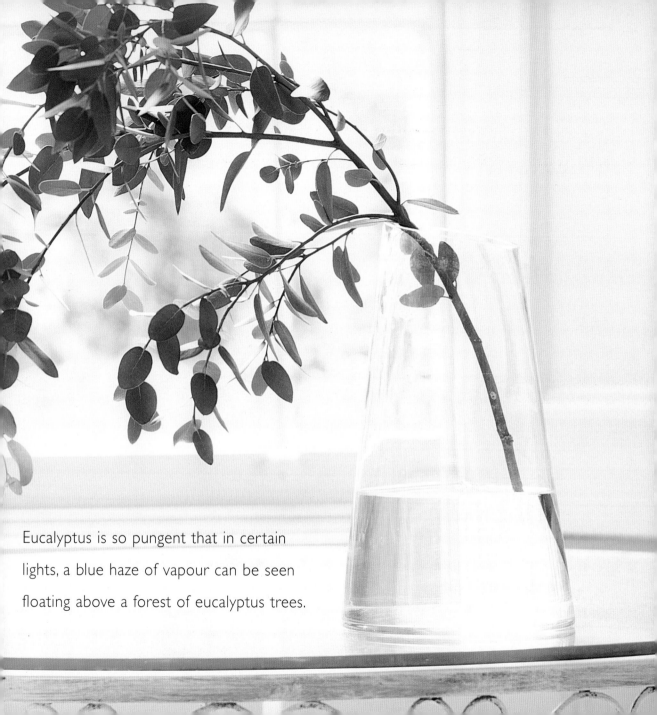

Eucalyptus is so pungent that in certain
lights, a blue haze of vapour can be seen
floating above a forest of eucalyptus trees.

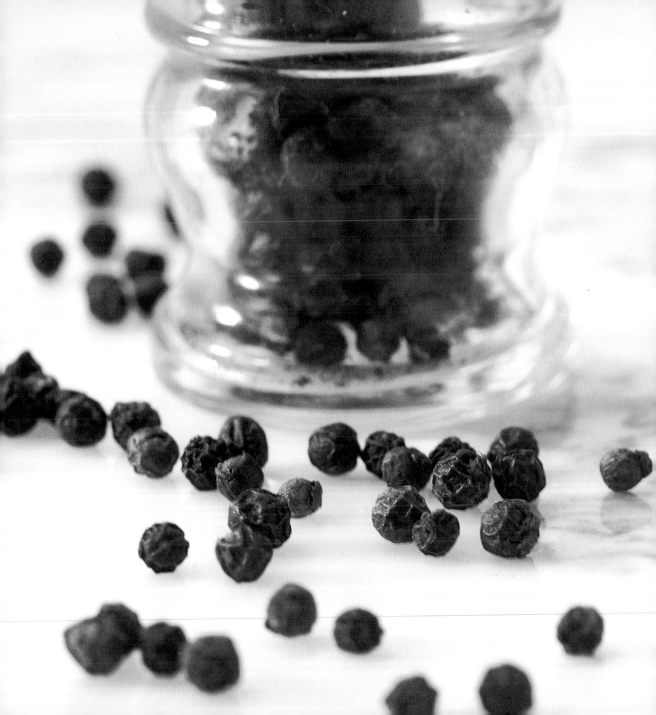

The use of pepper in cooking and medicine can be traced back over 4000 years. The essential oil is extracted from mature black pepper berries. It has a powerful aroma and is highly concentrated.

Black pepper oil is strong, fortifying and warming – much like the spice we know it as. These qualities make it suitable for improving a sluggish circulatory system. To massage cold hands and feet, rub them with a blend of 2 drops of black pepper oil and

Bathing in water that contains 2 drops of black pepper oil, 3 drops of frankincense oil and 1 drop of rose oil will also soothe tired, aching muscles. This particular remedy will clarify the mind, too.

Bruising responds well to black pepper. Soak a flannel in cool water with 2 drops of the oil, 2 drops of lavender oil and 1 drop of chamomile oil, then apply to the bruised area at regular intervals.

The pungent aroma of black pepper – released

black pepper *Piper nigrum*

The warm, soothing effect generated by black pepper makes it ideal for treating muscle aches, pains and strains. It can be used in a massage blend before and after exercise.

1 drop of geranium oil mixed with 5 ml (1 teaspoon) of vegetable, grapeseed or soya oil.

Aching muscles and stiff joints are common complaints suffered by sports enthusiasts and athletes. Use black pepper oil before and after exercise in a massage blend made with 3 drops of the oil and 1 drop of cypress and benzoin oil in 10 ml (1 dessertspoon) of vegetable oil. The deep, penetrating heat will warm the affected muscles.

when the oil is vaporized – with bergamot, lavender or lemon oil will help to overcome appetite loss by stimulating the digestive system. This same blend can also help to increase alertness.

As a precautionary note, because black pepper oil has stimulating and slightly diuretic properties, it is not recommended for use during pregnancy or by anyone suffering from high blood pressure. It can also irritate sensitive skin, so use in small doses.

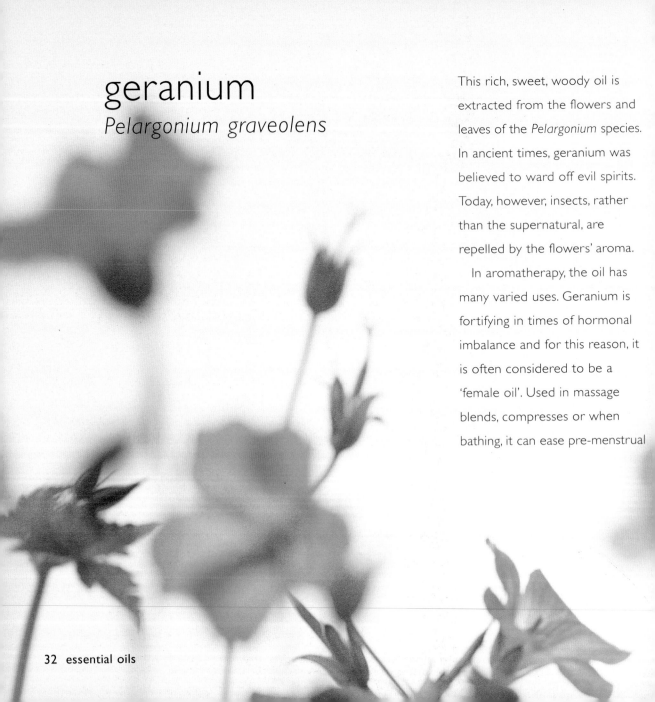

geranium
Pelargonium graveolens

This rich, sweet, woody oil is extracted from the flowers and leaves of the *Pelargonium* species. In ancient times, geranium was believed to ward off evil spirits. Today, however, insects, rather than the supernatural, are repelled by the flowers' aroma.

In aromatherapy, the oil has many varied uses. Geranium is fortifying in times of hormonal imbalance and for this reason, it is often considered to be a 'female oil'. Used in massage blends, compresses or when bathing, it can ease pre-menstrual tension (PMT) and menopausal problems. Combat PMT with a warm bath containing 3 drops of geranium oil, 2 drops of clary sage oil and 1 drop of orange oil.

Apply to the affected area, then cover with a towel and leave in place for as long as possible.

For fluctuating hormones, vaporizing a few drops of the oil function as an antidepressant.

When used in skincare treatments, geranium balances the secretion of sebum in the skin, making it particularly useful for oily and dry skin. It increases blood flow, giving tired skin a 'lift'. Blend 2 drops of geranium oil and 3 drops of mandarin oil with 10 ml of vegetable oil and massage onto areas which are susceptable to broken capillaries. (Use a weaker blend if applying to the face.)

Floral and exotic, and capable of provoking liberating, sensual emotions, geranium has a multitude of properties from regulator of hormonal swings to aphrodisiac.

Geranium's analgesic powers help to relieve painful periods and tender breasts. Soak a cloth in warm water with 3 drops each of geranium oil and lavender oil.

in a burner will help to create a harmonious and strengthening atmosphere. If you have an electric vaporizer, leave it on overnight. Geranium can also

Because of geranium's effect on the hormonal system, do not use the oil during pregnancy.

The name tea tree comes from the tea brewed from the leaves of *Melaleuca alternifolia* and drunk by Captain Cook during his exploration of Australia in the eighteenth century. Originally, the leaves were used by the Aborigines in natural remedies to treat wounds and illnesses.

Tea tree is the most researched of all the

Like lavender, tea tree is one of the few essential oils that can be applied neat. For spots, warts, verrucas, or infections under nails, dab a drop of the oil onto the affected area.

Tea tree can treat thrush and prevent it from reoccuring. When bathing, instead of using soap, add 6–10 drops of the oil to the water.

tea tree *Melaleuca alternifolia*

essential oils. Being a powerful antiseptic, antibacterial, antifungal and antiviral agent, tea tree's ability to fight infection is second to none – even its fragrance is 'medicinal'. No other essential oil possesses all of these properties. Tea tree is also the strongest, natural disinfectant, with studies showing it to be stronger than carbolic acid or phenol (chemical disinfectants). Fortunately, it is not poisonous to humans. All of these qualities make tea tree effective in treating athlete's foot, thrush, ringworm, insect bites, warts and verrucas, among other things. It can also be used to relieve and soothe itchy chickenpox.

Not only will this soothe the itchiness caused by thrush, but it will also deodorize and cleanse.

One other important aspect of tea tree is its stimulating action on the immune system. This makes it especially useful for colds, flu and debilitating illnesses such as glandular fever. Fight these infections by massaging a blend of 3 drops of tea tree oil and 1 drop of lavender oil mixed with 10 ml (1 dessertspoon) of vegetable oil onto the chest, back and neck.

To stop the spread of infectious illnesses, vaporize a few drops of tea tree oil, lemon oil and niaouli oil in a burner or electric vaporizer. This blend will also cleanse and freshen the air.

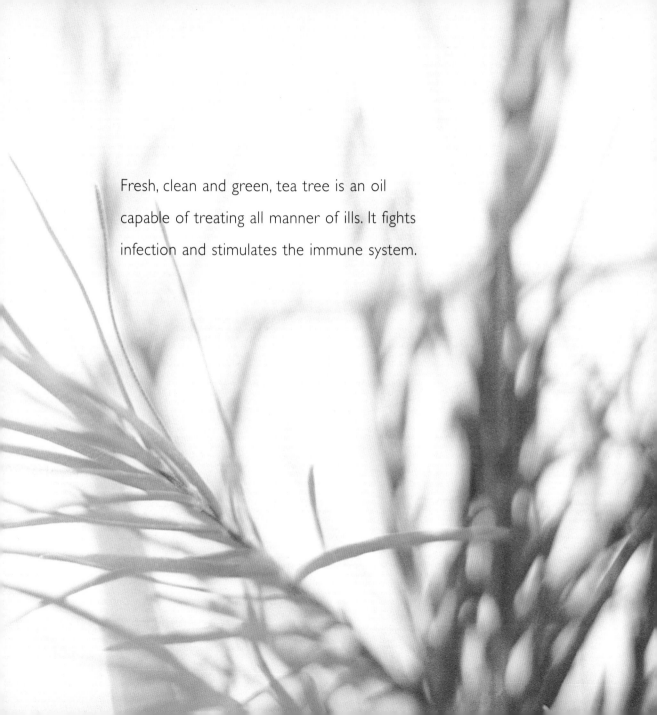

Fresh, clean and green, tea tree is an oil
capable of treating all manner of ills. It fights
infection and stimulates the immune system.

chamomile *Anthemis nobilis, Matricaria*

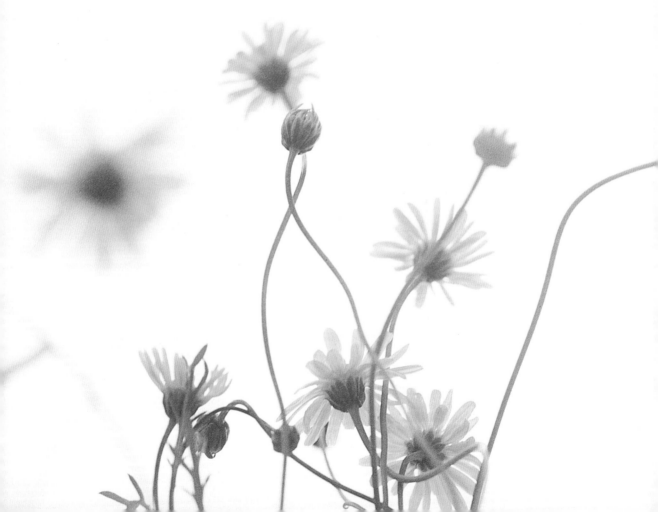

The oil from this delicate, daisy-like plant is valued for its ability to treat conditions where inflammation is present, whether internal or external. In its time, used in aromatherapy – Roman and German. The latter contains a higher level of azulin (an anti-inflammatory agent), but both have similar healing properties.

Chamomile: dedicated to the sun by the ancient Eygptians, described as a 'moon herb' by the Anglo-Saxons, and known as the 'plant physician' throughout the Mediterranean.

chamomile has been dedicated to the sun by the ancient Eygptians who used it to cure fevers; described as a 'moon herb' because of its cooling properties, and known as the 'plant physician', for its benefical effects on other plants when growing nearby.

There are many varieties of chamomile, but only two are

Chamomile is also an effective painkiller, making it is useful for muscular aches and pains, headaches, neuralgia – and just about any ailment or condition where a painkiller is needed.

A cold compress made by soaking a flannel in cool water with 3 drops of chamomile and lavender oil, and applied to the body will cool hot inflamed skin,

especially after sunburn, and will help lower a raised temperature.

Ease muscular pains, using a massage blend of 3 drops of chamomile oil, plus 1 drop each of lemongrass and lavender oil.

Chamomile has a profoundly calming and soothing effect on an emotional level, helping to relieve stress, depression and irritability.

A restless child or screaming baby can be calmed in a warm bath containing 1 drop of chamomile or lavender oil diluted in 5 ml (1 teaspoon) of vegetable oil or milk. This soothing bath blend is also good for period pains and pre-menstrual tension (PMT).

It is well known that chamomile tea can help disorders of the digestive and nervous system, but never take the oil internally.

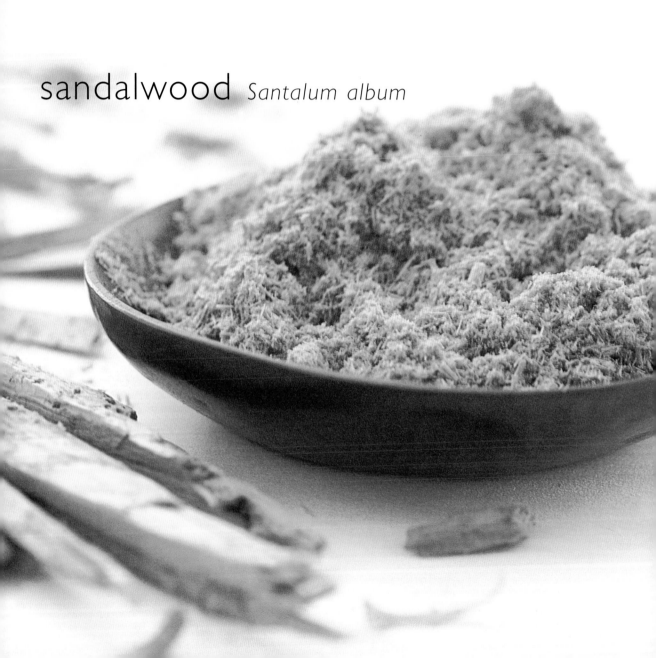

sandalwood *Santalum album*

This woody, sensuous oil from India is the oldest-known scent, its use spanning over 4000 years. Traditionally it was burned as incense in temples and was an important constituent in embalming.

Sandalwood's notable resistance to ant infestation has seen the trees harvested to near-extinction over the years to satisfy the building and furniture trade. Its oil is extracted from trees aged at least thirty, so it is not suprising that it is expensive.

In aromatherapy, sandalwood has a valuable role to play as a physical, spiritual and emotional healer. It is used regularly in the treatment of cystitis and other urinary infections because of its purifying and anti-inflammatory properties. A bath with 3 drops of sandalwood oil and 2 drops of tea tree and lemon oil will be soothing.

Although sandalwood has many uses, its best application is in skincare, being particulary effective for eczema, dry or chapped skin, razor rash and scalp conditions such as dandruff (see page 59).

Conversely, sandalwood's slightly astringent properties make it useful when added to a conditioner for greasy hair or to a neutral moisturizer for greasy skin.

Its musk-like fragrance has also earned a reputation for being a powerful aphrodisiac. To create a sexually charged atmosphere with candles, add 3 drops of sandalwood oil to the liquid wax as each candle burns.

To aid relaxation, a full-body massage using 2 drops each of sandalwood, chamomile and lavender oil diluted in 10 ml (1 dessertspoon) of vegetable oil will help to unburden feelings of anxiety.

Burned as an incense in Asian temples, sandalwood is gentle and sedating – a physical, spiritual and emotional healer. It is useful in skincare blends.

rose *Rosa centifolia, Rosa damascena*

Arguably the most celebrated of all floral essential oils, and strongly associated with romance and fertility. It has been described as the queen among essential oils.

A rose is the all-time symbol of love and purity. The ancient Roman ritual of scattering the bridal bed with scented rose petals to ensure a happy marriage is mirrored today with the throwing of confetti at weddings.

Only two varieties of rose are used to extract the oil and to produce the maximum yield the petals must be picked just after the morning dew has settled and distilled immediately. The oil can be extracted by steam distillation or enfleurage (see page 12). The oil produced by enfleurage is called an absolute and is expensive because it takes a vast amount of petals to produce just a tiny quantity.

Rose has very 'feminine' qualities and has an affinity with the reproductive system. It can be used to relieve pre-menstrual tension (PMT), regulate the menstrual cycle and ease menopausal problems. It can also have a significant effect on sexual problems such as frigidity in women and impotence in men, where emotional issues are also involved.

Rose is also a sedative and an antidepressant. It will soothe frayed emotions, calm nerves, cleanse the mind and lift depression. It has also proved invaluable in treating women suffering from post-natal depression. To restore tranquillity, vaporize 3 drops each of rose and lavender oil in a burner. This will also help to quell stomach upsets related to nervous tension.

Mature or wrinkled skin and broken veins beneath the skin's surface respond well to rose. For a nourishing face oil, mix 2 drops of the oil with 2 drops of neroli and jasmine oil diluted in 10 ml (1 dessertspoon) of jojoba oil. Store the mixture in a small dark bottle and massage onto the skin regularly as part of your skincare regime. It may be considered a luxury to use rose oil but the results are worth it.

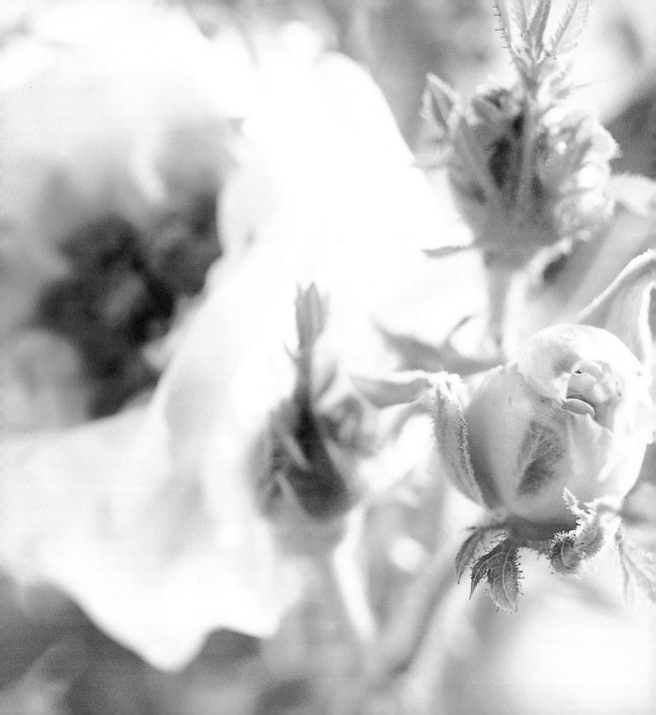

aromatherapy techniques
bathe, vaporize, compress, massage, reflexology...

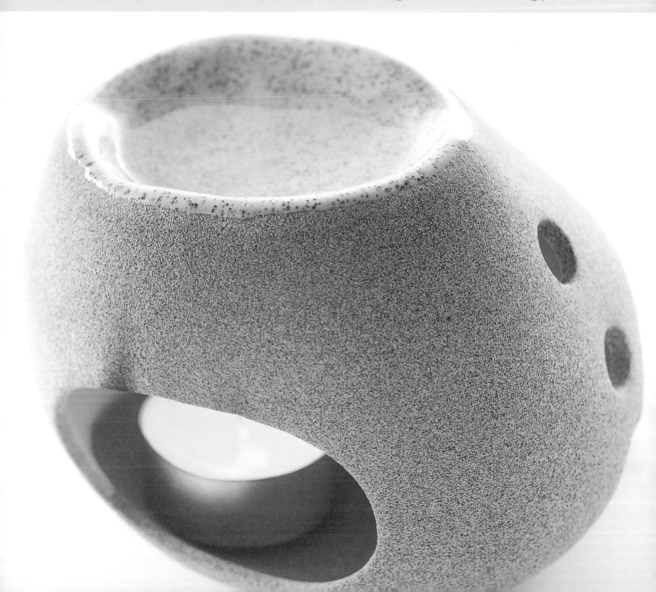

Essential oils can be used in many ways to deliver their therapeutic properties. But how you choose to use them is just as important as deciding which you need. Enjoying a massage or bath with essential oils are perhaps the best-known uses, but other applications like reflexology and vaporization are effective too. In this section you will also find a useful chart of common health problems and advice on which oils to use for their treatment. I also show how easy it is to use aromatherapy in your daily routine. Finally, to guide you in your endeavours, I give my favourite aromatherapy recipes and answer common concerns about using natural therapies. I hope that you learn more about essential oils so that as your confidence grows, you will be able to create and apply your own aromatherapy treatments.

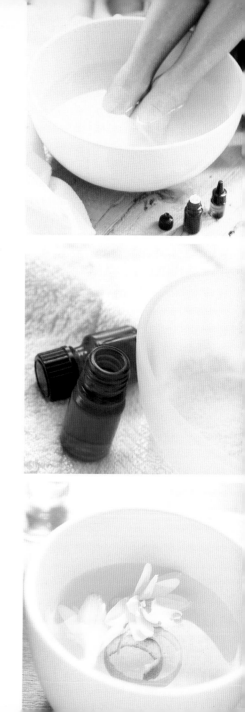

vaporization and inhalation

When exposed to the air, essential oils release their
therapeutic vapours into the atmosphere, and are
drawn into the body when the scent is inhaled.

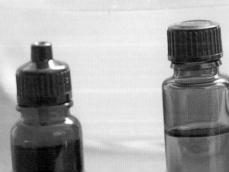
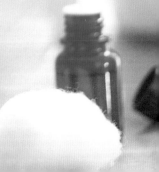

Vaporizing essential oils so they release their scent into the air, which is then inhaled, is a quick and effective way of delivering their benefits. Vaporized oils can also perfume, purify or freshen the air. Inhaling the oil's vapours can affect moods and emotions according to the properties of

below A bowl of scented water perched on a warm radiator will release pleasing aromas into the air.

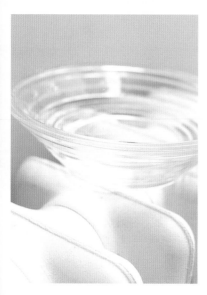

the oil being used. Just by smelling an oil you can tell if it will be stimulating or relaxing.

One of the best methods of vaporizing oils is in a ceramic burner. Add 4 drops of essential oil to water in the bowl and heat with a nightlight beneath.

A more expensive option is to use an electric vaporizer. It works like a standard burner, but without the heat of a naked flame. This makes it safer to use, which is especially important when children are nearby. Electric vaporizers can be left on during the night while you sleep. They have a thermostat, which allows the oils to burn safely and for longer at a low temperature.

Light bulb rings are made of porous ceramic, metal or fire-resistant card. They fit onto a light bulb and when the oil is added

and the light switched on, the heat from the bulb vaporizes the oil.

Essential oils may also be added to the melted wax of a lighted candle. This is more versatile than buying aromatherapy candles.

Vaporizing essential oils can be simpler still. Wring out a flannel which has been soaked in a bowl of water containing about 6 drops of essential oil, then put it on a radiator to dry and enjoy the fragrance. Alternatively, sprinkle oil onto a handkerchief and inhale the vapours periodically.

Steam inhalation is commonly associated with treating respiratory illnesses such as colds and flu. Add about 10 drops of pine, niaouli or eucalyptus oil to a bowl of hot water, then lean over the bowl and cover your head with a towel for about 10 minutes as you inhale.

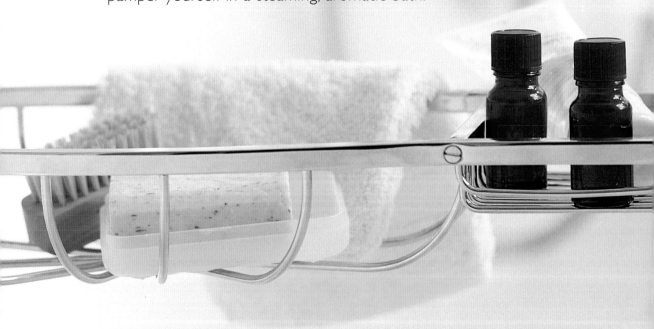

aromatic bathing

After a weary day at work – feeling worn out,
stressed, and in need of relaxation – unwind and
pamper yourself in a steaming, aromatic bath.

Bathing can be a pleasurable, highly relaxing experience and adding essential oils to your bathwater increases the benefits tenfold. As you bathe, you breathe in the oil's rich, aromatic vapours, which are carried in the steam, while the warmth of the water encourages your skin to absorb more of the oil.

For the perfect aromatic bath, do not exceed 10 drops of your favourite oil or blend of oils. Start by adding 6 drops and as you become familiar with their effects you can gradually increase the dosage. However, if you have sensitive skin you should not use more than 6 drops. Always add the oils after the water has been run and ensure that the water is not too hot or the oils will vaporize prematurely. Essential oils do not dissolve in water but instead float on the surface, so take care not to sit directly on them. Always add the oils at the tap end of the bath and thoroughly agitate the water to ensure an even distribution of oil. Citrus oils, especially, may sting the skin slightly if they are not properly dispersed.

For a luxurious, mosturizing bath, you can first blend your essential oils with a carrier oil (see pages 14–15). Grapeseed and almond oil are perfect for this and will leave your skin feeling soft and smooth. When bathing babies, first dilute a drop of lavender or chamomile oil in 5 ml (1 teaspoon) of milk or vegetable oil, then add to the water. For children aged two to six, do not exceed 4–6 drops of essential oil in the bath.

compresses and neat application

A fast and effective way to speed recovery from muscular pains and strains after a rigorous workout, and a treatment for bruises, headaches, insect bites, toothache, spots – and more.

An essential oil compress can be used to ease muscular aches, strains, bruises and headaches. It may be applied hot or cold depending on the type of pain or injury. In general, a hot compress is the most effective for treating muscular pains, such as backache, menstrual or stomach pains. It can also help to relieve rheumatic and arthritic pain, earache and toothache. For a pounding headache, insect bite, sprained muscle and other inflamed or swollen conditions that throb with pain and feel over-warm, use a cold compress. This will soothe the area and reduce swelling by constricting the blood supply to the site of the pain.

Compresses are quick and easy to apply. For a cold compress, soak a cloth in iced water to which chamomile and lavender oil have been added, then wring the cloth out and lay it on the affected area for at least fifteen minutes. Do the same to make a hot compress, but add black pepper and geranium oil to hot water instead of cold. (The water should be at a comfortable temperature.) A hot compress will cool quickly and must be replaced frequently.

In general, essential oils should not be applied neat to the skin as they can burn or cause mild irritation. However, lavender and tea tree oil are exceptions (see pages 22 and 34) and lemon oil may be used neat on warts and verrucas only. Ylang ylang, rose, jasmine, neroli and sandalwood oil may be used neat in tiny quantities as a perfume.

below Essential oils can be used to make a compress or blended with neutral creams, gels or lotions, then rubbed in. Use cotton wool balls to dab essential oils diluted with warm water onto the skin.

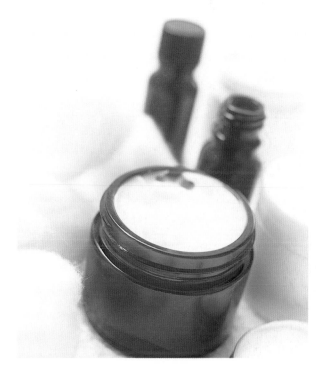

soothing massage

Massage – smoothing fragrant oil into tired muscles – is one of the most pleasurable ways to relax and unwind.

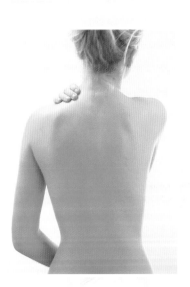

During a massage, taut muscles relax, tension is released and circulation is increased, giving a feeling of comfort and wellbeing. Even though professional masseurs undertake a complex study of anatomy, there is no reason why you can't give a massage to family, friends or a loved one at home. It is an age-old technique that is made even more powerful when combined with aromatherapy, since massaging a blend of essential oils into the skin is the most efficient way of delivering the oil's therapeutic properties. Different essential oils have different emotional effects. For example, when a sensuous essential oil such as ylang ylang is used, massage can bring two people closer together.

The environment for massage is important. Body temperature will drop during a massage, so make sure the room is warm and comfortable. To encourage relaxation, you can dim the lights or light candles, play soothing music and use warm towels.

Almost any part of the body can be massaged – back, legs, hands, feet, stomach, neck, shoulders and face all respond well to touch, though some areas are favoured more than others.

There are four basic massage techniques – effleurage, kneading, lymphatic drainage and friction – which can be used in combination to achieve a variety of effects.

Effleurage – a flowing, stroking motion, using one or two hands – should start and end a massage. Apply a range of pressures to relieve built-up tension.

Kneading is very good for aching muscles. Using the palms of your hands, gently manipulate the muscles as if you were kneading bread. Intersperse this motion with lighter strokes, but don't pinch or grab the skin.

A lymphatic drainage massage stimulates the lymph glands and is used to eliminate toxins from the body. This type of massage is excellent for treating cellulite. Make a detoxifying massage

blend (see page 58) and rub it on the legs and thighs where cellulite occurs. Gently pinch and roll sections of skin between your fingers, but don't be too rough.

A friction massage increases blood flow to the area being massaged. Use the thumbs in a circular motion on the skin. Again, try not to inflict pain – a massage is supposed to be enjoyable. Another way to create friction is to lubricate your hands with the massage blend, then rub your hands backwards and forwards quickly over the the skin to create heat.

A gentle facial massage in the evening is fantastic for relieving stress. Make a floral facial blend (see page 58) and work it into the skin following the fine lines and contours of the face and neck.

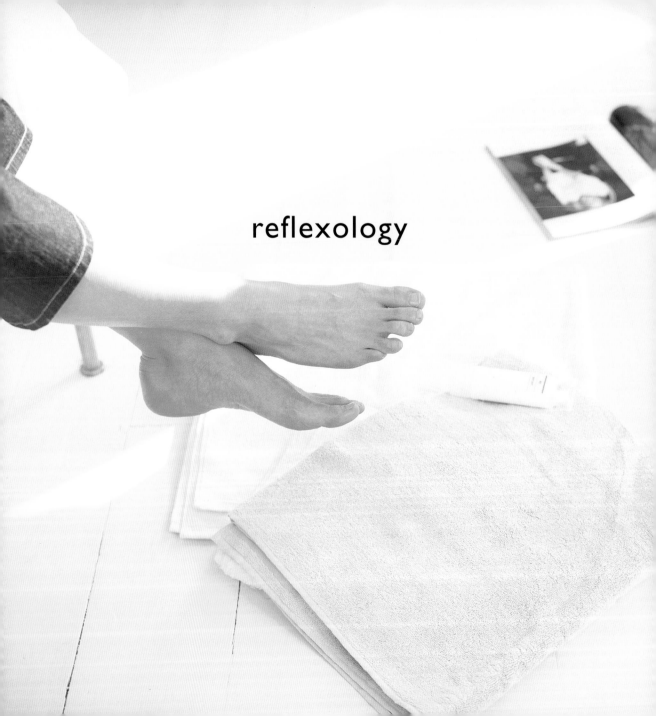

reflexology

A foot massage feels wonderful and when given using aromatherapy oils and reflexology techniques can also be very therapeutic. Reflexology is a form of foot massage that is used to diagnose and treat all manner of ills. It works on the principle that every part of the body is reflected in the feet.

A reflexologist will use his or her thumbs in a technique called 'walking' to locate and treat 'gritty' areas on the feet. These indicate an ailment in a corresponding part of the body. For example, if your big toe grinds when it is rotated, this could mean you have neck problems.

At home, you can simplify the treatment by using general massage movements (see pages 50–51). First soak your feet for about 10–15 minutes in a bowl of warm water containing 6 drops of blended essential oils. Choose from peppermint, tea tree, lemon, lavender and myrrh oil. Gently dry your feet. Using a foot massage blend (see page 58), work the oils into the feet with your hands, then cover one foot with a towel while you work on the other one. Pay particular attention to problem areas. For breathing complaints, concentrate on massaging the fleshy ball of the foot. Ease stomach and digestive problems by massaging under the instep. Massage the toes for ailments of the ears, eyes, nose and throat. To eliminate toxins from the body, massage between the toes. The big toe represents the head, with the spine running down the instep from big toe to heel, so massage these areas if you have a headache or backache. Massage around the ankles for disorders of the reproductive system. Once you have finished massaging one foot, wrap it in a towel and repeat the massage on

Your feet mirror the general wellbeing of your body. Treat them to a warm, aromatic foot bath and soothing massage.

the other foot. To finish, give each foot one final vigorous rub before slowing the movements down to gentle strokes. Finally, clasp the foot gently in your hands and hold this position for a few moments. Take a few deep breaths, then release your grip.

Hands can be massaged too. They have similar links to different parts of the body as the feet. Massaging hands and feet also promotes healthy skin and nails – and feels heavenly too.

remedies for common ailments

quick-reference chart for choosing and using appropriate essential oils

ailment	essential oils to use	methods of application
aches and pains	basil, benzoin, black pepper, chamomile, cinnamon, clove, cypress, ginger, juniper, lavender, marjoram, rosemary, thyme, ylang ylang	massage, compress, bath
acne	basil, bergamot, cedarwood, cypress, geranium, grapefruit, lavender, palmarosa, rose, tea tree	bath, massage
anxiety	bergamot, chamomile, fennel, geranium, grapefruit, jasmine, lavender, mandarin, marjoram, neroli, patchouli, petitgrain, pine, rose, rosewood, sandalwood, orange, vetivert, ylang ylang	bath, massage, vaporization, inhalation
asthma	chamomile, frankincense, myrtle, myrrh, pine	bath, massage, vaporization, inhalation
athlete's foot	lavender, lemon, myrrh, tea tree	bath, neat application
chest problems	benzoin, frankincense, myrtle, myrrh, niaouli, pine, rosemary, tea tree, thyme	bath, massage, vaporization, inhalation
chilblains	benzoin, black pepper, cedarwood, ginger, juniper, marjoram, thyme	massage, bath, compress
colds and flu	basil, benzoin, black pepper, cinnamon, eucalyptus, ginger, lavender, lemon, myrtle, niaouli, peppermint, pine, tea tree, thyme	bath, massage, vaporization, inhalation
constipation	black pepper, clary sage, cypress, eucalyptus, peppermint, rosemary	massage, bath, compress
cramp	chamomile, lavender, marjoram, sandalwood, vetivert	massage, bath, compress
cystitis	chamomile, lavender, tea tree, geranium, pine, sandalwood	bath, massage, compress
dandruff	cedarwood, lavender, lemongrass, sandalwood	scalp massage, rinse
depression	bergamot, clary sage, geranium, grapefruit, jasmine, lavender, lemon, mandarin, neroli, rose, orange, ylang ylang	bath, massage, vaporization, inhalation
diarrhoea	chamomile, lavender, rose, neroli	bath, massage, compress
eczema	benzoin, chamomile, lavender, myrrh, sandalwood, vetivert	bath, massage

ailment	essential oils to use	methods of application
fluid retention	black pepper, cypress, juniper	massage, bath
hay fever	bergamot, cedarwood, chamomile, eucalyptus, geranium, lavender, lemongrass, myrtle, pine, rose, rosemary, rosewood, ylang ylang	bath, massage, vaporization, inhalation
headaches	chamomile, lavender, lemongrass, peppermint, rosewood	vaporization, inhalation, bath, massage
headlice	bergamot, eucalyptus, geranium, lavender, lemon, tea tree	scalp massage, rinse
herpes	chamomile, lavender, myrrh, tea tree	bath, massage, compress, neat application
high blood pressure	bergamot, chamomile, fennel, frankincense, lavender, mandarin, marjoram, neroli, rose, sandalwood, vetivert, ylang ylang	massage, bath, vaporization, inhalation
indigestion	dill, fennel, parsley, peppermint, mandarin	massage, inhalation
menstrual problems	black pepper, chamomile, clary sage, geranium, jasmine, lavender, marjoram, neroli, rose	bath, massage, compress, vaporization, inhalation
nausea	bergamot, black pepper, chamomile, fennel, ginger, grapefruit, lavender, mandarin, orange, peppermint, rosewood	bath, inhalation, vaporization
post-natal depression	bergamot, chamomile, clary sage, fennel, frankincense, geranium, grapefruit, jasmine, lavender, lemon, neroli, orange, petitgrain, rose, sandalwood, ylang ylang	bath, massage, vaporization, inhalation
sinusitis	chamomile, eucalyptus, lavender, lemon, lemongrass, myrtle, niaouli, peppermint, pine, tea tree	bath, massage, inhalation, vaporization
sprains	chamomile, lavender	massage, compress, bath
stress	bergamot, chamomile, frankincense, geranium, grapefruit, jasmine, lavender, mandarin, marjoram, neroli, orange, patchouli, petitgrain, pine, rose, rosewood, sandalwood, vetivert, ylang ylang	massage, bath, vaporization, inhalation
stretch marks	mandarin, neroli, rose	bath, massage
throat infections	basil, benzoin, black pepper, cinnamon, eucalyptus, lavender, lemon, myrtle, niaouli, peppermint, pine, sandalwood, tea tree	bath, massage, vaporization, inhalation, compress
thrush	lavender, tea tree, myrrh	bath, cool compress

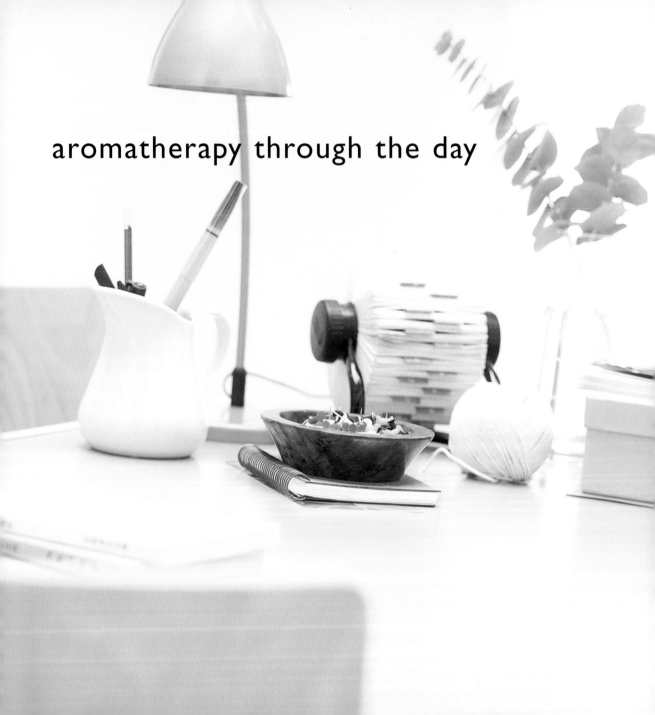
aromatherapy through the day

Morning, noon or night, essential oils work their magic effortlessly. Here are a few examples of when and how to use them.

EARLY MORNING Stimulating essential oils such as lemon, grapefruit or rosemary are perfect for clearing the morning fuzz when you wake up. Inhale the aroma from one or a blend of these oils to awaken your senses.

BATHE Add a few drops of bergamot oil to your bathwater or the shower floor. The vapours will put you in a good frame of mind ready for the day ahead.

TRAVEL Scent a handkerchief with drops of rosewood or lemongrass oil, then carry it with you on your daily travels. Inhaling the vapours periodically will enable you to arrive at your destination calm and refreshed.

AT WORK Cedarwood and peppermint oil are uplifting. Put 1–2 drops of the oil on a cloth and lay it on top of your computer. The gentle heat from the machine will diffuse the oil's aroma and keep you alert all day.

AT HOME Wipe surfaces with lemon or lavender-scented water to impart fragrance as well as neutralize microbes. In the bathroom, a pine-scented bath mat will keep the atmosphere fresh. For other rooms, a wet cloth scented with petitgrain and orange oil left to dry on a radiator will produce a relaxing effect.

STUDYING Rosemary oil promotes concentration. Lightly scent a handkerchief with a few drops of the oil and inhale the vapours from time to time as you work.

EVENING Time to change gear and slow down after a busy day. Vaporize neroli or jasmine oil to create a luxurious atmosphere to reward and pamper yourself.

PARTY Clary sage is supposed to make you feel irresistible. If you are getting ready to go out, use a few drops of the oil in your bathwater or add it to a hair rinse. If you are pregnant or have a medical condition, use neroli oil instead. It is subtle but just as effective.

ENTICE Nothing is more sensuous than a massage with essential oils. Blend ylang ylang and rose oils – reputed aphrodisiacs – with carrier oils for pure romance.

RELAX To promote restful slumber and relaxation in the evening, vaporize sandalwood or patchouli oil in the molten wax of a burning candle. Prepare children for bedtime by adding chamomile, myrtle or lavender oil to their bathwater. These oils are perfect for calming and relaxing tired bodies and minds, and will ensure youngsters are comfortable, cosy, and above all, sleepy.

SLEEP Frankincense promotes deep breathing, while marjoram is relaxing. Added to an electric vaporizer, the oils encourage sleep and will continue to work through the night. Keep the aroma subtle for a good night's sleep.

aromatherapy recipes for wellbeing

fragrant, healing blends to restore and maintain physical and mental health

ACHES AND PAINS

Help relieve aches and pains in joints and muscles.

1 drop of black pepper oil

1 drop of cypress oil

1 drop of lavender oil

1 drop of benzoin oil

Blend the oils with 10 ml of a carrier, such as grapeseed oil, neutral cream or lotion. Massage into the skin or add to bathwater. Alternatively, omit the carrier and vaporize the essential oils.

CIRCULATION

Promote a healthy circulation.

2 drops of juniper oil

2 drops of cypress oil

1 drop of benzoin oil

Mix the oils with 10 ml of a carrier, such as grapeseed oil, neutral cream or lotion, and use for massage or in bathing.

DETOXIFYING BLEND

Spring clean your body. To help eliminate toxins, use this blend daily for massage or in bathing.

2 drops of rosemary oil

1 drop of cypress oil

1 drop of juniper oil

1 drop of lemon oil

Blend the oils with 10 ml of a carrier, such as grapeseed oil, neutral cream or lotion.

FACIAL MASSAGE BLEND

Feed and nourish your face and neck with this floral oil blend.

1 drop of jasmine oil

1 drop of rose oil

1 drop of ylang ylang oil

1 drop of lavender oil

5 ml of grapeseed oil

5 ml of jojoba oil

Mix the oils and gently massage on your face and neck daily.

FOOT BATH/MASSAGE BLEND

Give your feet a reflexology treatment, using this blend.

2 drops of lavender oil

1 drop of lemon oil

1 drop of tea tree oil

1 drop of peppermint oil

Blend the oils with 10 ml of a carrier such as grapeseed oil and add to a foot bath or use to massage your feet. (See page 53.)

HEADLICE

After using this insect-repellent blend, lice will lose their grip on the hair and can be combed out.

1 drop of lemon oil

1 drop of tea tree oil

1 drop of geranium oil

1 drop of lavender oil

1 drop of eucalyptus oil

Blend the oils with 10 ml of grapeseed oil then massage into your scalp and hair. Rinse out, then wash and dry your hair as normal. Repeat the treatment after three days.

INSOMNIA

Encourage deep, restful sleep with this ultra-soporific blend.

2 drops of frankincense oil

1 drop of lavender oil

1 drop of marjoram oil

1 drop of sandalwood oil

Vaporize the oils or mix them with 10 ml of a carrier and use for massage or in bathing.

PREGNANCY: LABOUR PAINS

A fragrant blend to help soothe pain and promote calm breathing during strong contractions.

2 drops of frankincense oil

1 drop of mandarin oil

1 drop of lemon oil

1 drop of grapefruit oil

Vaporize the oils or blend them with 10 ml of grapeseed oil and use for massage or add to a bath.

SCALP CONDITIONER

For dry and flaky scalp conditions such as dandruff, massage this condtioning blend into your scalp.

1 drop of cedarwood oil

1 drop of sandalwood oil

1 drop of benzoin oil

1 drop of lemongrass oil

1 drop of rosemary oil

Blend the oils with 10 ml of grapeseed oil then massage into your scalp. Rinse, then wash and dry your hair as normal. Repeat this treatment once a week.

STRESS

A blend to help you unwind and promote a relaxed state of mind.

2 drops of lavender oil

2 drops of bergamot oil

1 drop of vetivert oil

Blend the oils with 10 ml of a carrier, such as grapeseed oil, neutral cream or lotion. Rub into the skin or add to a bath. Alternatively, omit the carrier and vaporize the essential oils.

your questions answered

Newcomers to aromatherapy face similar dilemmas when deciding what essential oils to use safely and effectively. These are a few of the questions that I am most often asked.

CAN I USE ESSENTIAL OILS IF I AM PREGNANT?

Yes you can, but avoid oils that have diuretic properties, such as juniper and cypress. Oils that raise or lower blood pressure, such as black pepper, and geranium which may affect hormone levels, should not be used. Mandarin oil is the best oil to use during pregnancy because its effect is mild and gentle (see page 26). As a rule, use floral or fruit essential oils to relax and to keep your skin in good condition. See pages 18–21 for suitable oils. Consult your doctor before using any essential oil.

CAN I USE ESSENTIAL OILS FOR MY BABY?

Chamomile and lavender oil are the only essential oils gentle enough for newborn babies (see pages 22 and 36). Both oils are calming and may be vaporized if your baby is restless or has difficulty sleeping. Alternatively, dilute 1–2 drops of the oils in 10 ml of grapeseed oil for massage or in 5 ml of milk, to add to bathwater. Once your baby is two weeks old, dill oil may be used, as above, to ease trapped wind and myrtle oil to treat snuffles. Always dilute the oils before use.

I HAVE SENSITIVE SKIN. CAN I USE ESSENTIAL OILS?

Many commercial perfumes and skincare products contain potential irritants, such as detergent, alcohol, mineral oil or colorants. Essential oils are totally natural and a few, such as chamomile and mandarin, may be used diluted on sensitive skin. Dilute essential oils before use and carry out a patch test first (see page 15). Babies and the eldery have delicate skin, so they should never use essential oils neat. Instead, dilute the oils in a carrier oil for massage or in 5 ml (1 teaspoon) of milk, to add to bathwater.

IS AROMATHERAPY GOOD FOR HIGH BLOOD PRESSURE?

Yes, but avoid stimulating oils such as black pepper, clary sage, juniper, cinnamon and ginger. Oils that calm or sedate, such as chamomile, rose and vetivert will be safe and pleasurable to use.

I SUFFER FROM EPILEPSY. CAN I USE ESSENTIAL OILS?

Yes, but avoid stimulating oils, such as those listed above.

WILL ESSENTIAL OILS WARD OFF INSECTS?

Citronella, lemon, lavender and geranium are natural insect repellents. Vaporize any of these oils in an oil burner, or scent a handkerchief with them and store in a wardrobe or drawer to protect clothing and household linen from moths. This will also impart a lovely fragrance, freshening the air in the room.

CAN I USE ESSENTIAL OILS TO TREAT HEADLICE?

Mix suitable oils to make a conditioning massage blend (see page 58). After use, lice will lose their grip on the hair and can be combed out. The blend will also help keep lice away. Repeat the treatment after three days.

CAN I USE ESSENTIAL OILS ON OPEN WOUNDS?

Tea tree oil is one of the very few essential oils that can be used neat as an antiseptic on broken skin. For serious wounds always consult your doctor.

HOW LONG DO ESSENTIAL OILS STAY IN THE BODY AND WHEN DO THEIR EFFECTS WEAR OFF?

Essential oils remain in the body for up to three days, after which they are metabolized and excreted. Some oils have an instantaneous effect on the mind and body, while others release their power over time, triggering a healing process that can continue for days or weeks.

ARE ESSENTIAL OILS SUITABLE FOR THE ELDERLY?

Essential oils are highly potent substances and must be used with care and respect. For the frail, avoid stimulating oils such as clary sage and sedating oils like marjoram. When using other essential oils, halve the quantities recommended in this book. If the elderly person is in good health no special precautions should be necessary.

DOES AROMATHERAPY HAVE A PLACE ALONGSIDE ORTHODOX AND HOMEOPATHIC MEDICINE?

Yes, but you should consult your doctor if you are on strong medication. Peppermint and ginger oils are not recommended with homeopathic medicines. Essential oils can help to treat ailments but they are not a substitute for prescribed medication.

CAN ESSENTIAL OILS HELP ME SLEEP?

Vaporizing frankincense, marjoram, sandalwood or neroli oil before you go to bed will encourage deep breathing and relaxation. The sedating effects can be continued through the night if you use the oils in an electric vaporizer. Soaking in a warm bath containing a few drops of essential oil such as lavender or neroli oil, can also help you to relax and unwind before bedtime.

WHAT SHOULD I DO IF I SWALLOW AN ESSENTIAL OIL?

If more than 1 or 2 drops of essential oil are swallowed, contact your doctor immediately and drink plenty of water or milk to dilute the oil. Prevention is better than cure. Never take any essential oil internally.

WHAT IF AN ESSENTIAL OIL GETS IN MY EYES?

Act quickly. Rinse your eyes thoroughly with milk. This will dissolve the oil and take away its sting. If symptoms persist, consult your doctor.

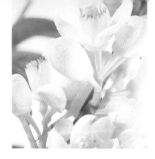

useful addresses

SUPPLIERS OF ESSENTIAL OILS AND ASSOCIATED PRODUCTS

Cariad Ltd
104 Bancroft
Hitchin
Hertfordshire, SG5 1LY
Tel: 01462 443518
(mail order and advice)
Fax: 01462 443516
info@cariad.co.uk
www.cariad.co.uk
Manufacturer, supplier and distributor of an extensive range of top-quality essential oils, carrier oils, creams, gels, flower waters and gifts. Phone for your nearest stockist.

Enata
11 Kings Drive
Thames Ditton
Surrey, KT7 0TH
Tel: 020 8339 0696
Fax: 020 8339 0811
info@enata.co.uk
www.enata.co.uk
Bespoke perfumery service and supplier of elite therapists.

The Fragrant Earth Co. Ltd
Orchard Court
Magdalene Street
Glastonbury
Somerset, BA6 9EW
Tel: 01458 831216
www.fragrant-earth.com
Mail order suppliers of organic absolutes, essential oils and blended oils and associated products, including books.

Micheline Arcier
Aromatherapy
7 William Street
London, SW1X 9HL
Tel: 020 7235 3545
Mail order suppliers of essential oils and blended massage oils. Therapists offer treatments in reflexology, massage and aromatherapy.

PROFESSIONAL BODIES AND ORGANIZATIONS

Federation of Holistic
Therapists
3rd Floor
Eastleigh House
Upper Market Street
Eastleigh
Hampshire, SO50 9FD
Tel: 01703 488 900

International Federation of
Aromatherapists (IFA)
Stamford House
182 Chiswick High Road
London, W4 1PP
Tel: 020 8742 2605
Fax: 020 8742 2606
www.ifaroma.org

International Federation
of Essential Oils and
Aroma Trades
130 Wigmore Street
London, W1H 9FE
Tel: 020 7935 2143

International Society of
Professional Aromatherapists
Hinkley & District Hospital
and Health Centre
The Annexe
Mount Road
Hinkley
Leics, LE10 1AG
Tel: 01455 637 987

Association of Reflexologists
7 Old Gloucester Street
London, WC1N 3XX
Tel: 0990 673320

TRAINING COURSES

ITEC
4 Heathfield Terrace
Chiswick
London, W4 4JE
Tel: 020 8994 4141
Fax: 020 8994 7880
info@itecworld.co.uk
www.itecworld.co.uk
International Therapy Examination Council who have a list of accredited colleges in the UK and internationally too.

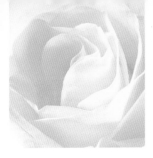

acknowledgements

I would like to thank my husband Haydn, for always being there, and for helping to turn my erratic word processing into something the publisher could read. I would also like to dedicate this book to my children Megan and Elliot, so that they will always know and understand what I do. Next I want to thank Mum, Dad and all my family in England, Wales and Italy for all their support.

Thank you to all at Cariad for being so patient while I took valuable time out to write this book, for your constant encouragement and for keeping everything running so smoothly at the office during my absence.

To Anne Ryland and her fantastic team at Ryland Peters & Small – thank you for making *The Essence of Aromatherapy* happen.

Many thanks to Stephen Hughes for his time and advice, and for sharing – freely and amusingly – his extensive knowledge of the industry. Also, thanks to James Plant at Garson's Farm for helping me to track down the plants that were photographed in the book.

And finally, thank you to David Montgomery for his beautiful photography.

Index